STOP THE CLOCK:

CAN WE LIVE LONGER

BY REVERSING AGING PROCESS?

BY RACHITA KUMAR

Disclaimer

The advice contained in this material might not be suitable for everyone. The author obtained the information from sources believed to be reliable and from his own personal experience, but he neither implies nor intends any guarantee of accuracy.

The author, publisher and distributors never give legal, accounting, medical or any other type of professional advice. The reader must always seek those services from competent professionals that can review their own particular circumstances.

The author, publisher and distributors particularly disclaim any liability, loss, or risk taken by individuals who directly or indirectly act on the information contained herein. All readers must accept full responsibility for their use of this material.

Table of Contents

INTRODUCTION

"Youth would be an ideal state if it came a little later
in life." - *Herbert Asquith*

---

*T*he question '*How to stop the aging
processes?*' has engaged the human mind
since inception of recorded civilization. Man
has tried to find solution in mythology, religion, yoga
and of late in scientific breakthrough. We hate growing
old. Therefore, as we move up in age, the thought of
retaining our youth gets intensified. It is the natural
state of things.

According to Greek mythology, Aurora, the goddess
of dawn fell in love with a mortal young man
named Tithonus. When Zeus, the king of Gods granted
Aurora a wish for her lover, she asked for his
immortality but, in haste, she forgot to ask for his
eternal youth. Consequently, he grew old and as years
passed by, Tithonus gradually lost his strength and
vigor. Aurora therefore doomed Tithonus to a life of
eternal old age.

The Greek mythology has always mesmerized me.
The Greeks have dished out some very important and
eternal truth that man has to face in their daily life in

the form of stories. They might have gifted us their fascinating imaginary stories without even knowing how important and relevant those stories might turn out to be. The story ofTithonus and Aurora is just an example. This very fascinating and romantic story depicts the greatest problem faced by mankind - aging.

Greeks considered themselves to be the children of God. Therefore, they tried to understand the eternal life of God by their mortal sight. They thought that the eternal life of God had similar mortal phases. And in the process, they blended mortal ideas with their spiritual beliefs. This is probably the reason why Aurora had to request Zeus to grant immortality for her perpetual lover.

The Greeks had it almost right, but it is still wrong. Therefore, what they did was no other than an imitation of the truth. Imitation occurs only for valuable things. Things that are not valuable are never imitated. For instance, monopoly money is never imitated as it is valueless. US currency on the other hand has often been imitated for its high value. Only the valuable things are worth imitating. Truth is always worth imitating for it has high importance and value.

I guess one has to be quite careful with what one asks for. We should therefore always be careful about what we ask for. Aurora asked for Tithonus' immortality so that she never loses him to death. She got all that she wanted. But Tithonus had to suffer for her actions and lead a painfully miserable life that would never come to an end.

In our quest for finding immortality we should not be misled by so many unproven theories on anti-aging and suffer the consequences as aptly brought out in the mythological story above.

During the last century medical science managed to double the life span of human species mainly due to prevention of diseases. Will the trend continue in future? Will we manage to double the human life again in this century? Few renowned scientists are already saying that babies have been born who will live beyond 150 years. Is there any truth in these predictions?

The purpose of this book is to examine facts from fiction as to what is happening in the field of anti-aging. It is important because it has huge implications for us as individuals and society as a whole.

Chapter 1 - Why we Age - Stress and Immune Response, Stress and Inflammation

The study of aging is called "Gerontology". The term is derived from the Greek words *'geron'* meaning old man, and *'logy'* meaning study. Gerontology discovers the social, biological and psychological changes in people as they age. This is a comparatively new branch of science that has amazingly developed in the last 30 years. The scientists of gerontology are trying to find the single reason behind aging. Their primary question to which gerontologists are trying to find an answer to is, "Is aging naturally programmed into a living body" or "Is it the result of damages that are accumulated over time"?

According to the theories, aging is a complex interaction of genetics, chemistry, psychology and behavior. Through this book, we will have a wider look at the following theories of aging:

1. The human body follows a certain biological timeline and is designed to age with time.

2. Certain predetermined genes switch on and off with time and cause aging.

3. Certain changes in the hormonal structures and amount of secretion control and cause aging.

4. The immune system declines over time for various reasons and leaves the body exposed to diseases.

5. Aging might also be caused by the damages incurred by the environment on our body.

6. Daily wear and tear of cells and tissues in the body cause aging.

7. The faster a living organism metabolizes oxygen, the shorter life it lives.

8. Body process is slowed down due to the accumulation of cross-linked protein that results in aging.

9. Free radicals can damage cells and overshadow their function and cause aging.

10. Genetic change because of cell malfunctioning can also cause aging.

Genetics and Aging

Our genes play an important role in aging. Researchers have found that, the lifespan of certain organisms can almost be doubled by adjusting their genes. Though the aptness of such experiments for human beings is not known, researchers believe that genetics justify about 35% variations in aging among people. They believe that the potential lifespan of an individual is usually determined at the moment of conception. This explains why identical twins, whose genes are exactly the same, have almost the same lifespan.

1. Longevity genes: These are the special beneficiary genes that help a person to live longer. For example, they help in metabolizing cholesterol and thereby reduce the risk of heart disease.

2. Cell Senescence: It is the process that deteriorates the health and function of cells over time.

3. Telomeres: These structures are located at the end of DNA. They protect the chromosomes during cell division and get depleted in the process. After about 50 such cell divisions, these telomeres become so small that they are unable to duplicate any further. This leads to cellular dysfunction and results to aging and death.

4. Stem Cells: These cells can convert themselves into any kind of cell and repair the damages caused by aging.

Biochemistry

Our body unceasingly undergoes complex biochemical reactions, no matter what genes we have inherited. Some of these reactions can cause damage in the body and result in aging. A close study of these complex reactions help researchers in understanding the various changes incurred by the body as it ages. Some important concepts of the theory of biochemistry are;

1. Free Radicals - Eating, drinking and breathing in daily life forms free-radicals or unstable oxygen molecules from the energy production cycles. These molecules attack the structure of cell membranes and create toxic metabolic wastes that disturb DNA, RNA and protein synthesis and damage cells.

2. Protein Cross-Linking – When there is excess glucose in the blood, the glucose molecules are cross-linked to protein. These molecules don't function properly. When enough cross-linked molecules accumulate in a specific tissue, these tissues stiffen and fail to function efficiently.

3. DNA repair - DNA is the blueprint of the life we inherit from our parents. We are born with a unique code that predetermines the physical and

mental functioning of our body and regulate the rate at which we age. As we mature the systems in our body that repair DNA lose their effectiveness that results in aging.

4. Heat shock Proteins - The heat shock proteins are also called stress proteins. They stabilize partially unfolded proteins and control stress.

5. Hormones - The hypothalamus ob the brain controls various chain-reactions and instruct organs and glands to release their hormones. But as we grow old the hypothalamus loses its ability to instruct and the receptors. Therefore the secretion of many hormones decline and lose their effectiveness.

Body Systems

Our body undergoes various changes with age. These changes in the organs and systems in our body adjust and modify our immunity to different diseases. The reasons behind such changes, though necessary, have not yet been understood by researchers. Some important effects of aging on our organs body system are,

1. Heart - As we age, the muscles of the heart thicken along with the thickening of arteries. This

lowers the maximum pumping rate of the heart and leads to extremely low diastolic blood pressure.

2. Immune system – As we age, the T-cells in our body take a longer time to rejuvenate. This lowers their capability to function thereby exposing them to diseases.

3. Arteries – The arteries in body tend to harden as we age. This makes it difficult for the heart to pump blood through them.

4. Lungs – As a person ages, the working capacity of the lungs continues decreasing. By the time a person is 70 years old, the functioning ability of the lungs declines by 40%

5. Brain – Some connections between nerve cells appear to be subdued or reduced in efficiency as the brain matures.

6. Kidneys – The efficiency of the kidneys reduce as a person grows old. They become less efficient in cleaning the waste products from blood.

7. Bladder – As a person ages, the tissues decay and the total capacity of the bladder decreases.

8. Body fat and aging – The body fat level keeps on rising as a person matures. However, once he crosses middle age it is customary for body fat to decrease. Also, the fat sinks deeper into the body as we age.

9. Muscle – The strength and tonicity of muscles goes down by about 22% by the time a person reaches the age of 70. Nevertheless the process of losing strength can be slackened by regular exercise.

10. Bone – Our bones start losing consistency at the age of 35. This process can also be slowed down by walking, running and resistance training.

11. Eyes – People usually experience difficulty in seeing minute details after the age of 40.

12. Ear – The ability to hear high frequency sounds decrease as a person matures with age.

Behavioral Factors

We can change the way we age modifying our behavior.

- We can minimize the damage caused by free radicals by eating food that is rich in antioxidants.
- Loss in strength of muscles and bones can be limited by regular exercise.

- Cholesterol levels can be kept under control by brisk-walking and consuming foods rich in fiber. This will slow down the hardening of arteries and protect the heart.
- We can retain the sharpness of brain and keep it active by practicing mental fitness.
- Leading a healthy life and maintaining a healthy calorie-restricted diet can increase life by 40%
- Positive thinking and having a positive approach towards life can also increase life by approximately 7.5 years.

Is Aging Programmed?

According to the programmed theory of aging, growing old is an inherent and inseparable part of biology. It has been innately programmed into our body system and connected to the three main systems of our body – endocrine system, immune system and genetics.

The evidence that supports this theory is that there is not much variation in the lifespan of a certain species. This implies that, we are all programmed to age and die after a certain predetermined period of time.

Is Body a Machine?

Though human body is not a machine, we often tend to compare them to each other. Unlike a machine it is not possible for us to manually activate or deactivate a muscle or a system in our body according to our wish. Moreover, human body constantly repairs and replaces cells accordingly so that every 7 years about 90% cells in our body are rejuvenated. The human body is an amazing and vigorous system. We can understand its function only if we forget machines and concentrate on living beings.

Aging is About Evolution, Not Biology

Evolution of aging aims to explain why all living beings weaken and die with age. The question most frequently arises here is - "should the human body "wear out?" It has already been declared that, the human body can recreate and regenerate itself. Time is possibly a major factor that plays an important role in maturing the human body. But there must be additional factors at play that cause the unavoidable consequences of aging. This question leads us to the programmed theory of aging that considers aging and death to be two indispensable parts of evolution but disagree to accept it as a part of biology. Every species require a genetic capacity for aging and death otherwise it would not be forced to replicate in order to exist. Species would simply continue existing till something wiped them out completely. If biological individuals have an eternal existence, there would be no evolution at all.

Programmed Aging

According to this theory, Aging is innately programmed in an organism and is not the outcome of environmental factor or wear and tear. Therefore, aging and death are not the outcome of any kind of exposure to environment but is a programmed response to an instinctive and indispensable part of genetics. The evidence shows that there is not much of variation in lifespan among organisms of the same species. Elephants die around the age of 70, spider monkeys die around 25, and human beings die around the age of 80. Though modifications in diet and lifestyle can increase the quality an individual's life span but general lifespan within species is moderately invariant. In other words, proper nutrition and healthy habits stimulates a high quality of life but does not promise quantity of life. If aging were due to "wear and tear" there would be to a greater extent variation in lifespan within the same species.

How do Hormones affect Aging?

The most significant aspect of aging are the modifications brought about in the body by the endocrine system. Many hormones decline and become less effective as we age. The most important hormonal changes are the ones that take place in estrogen before and after menopause in women. Testosterone levels also decrease in men, but not as drastically as estrogen in women and never dropping below "normal" levels.

In order to establish and prove this theory, researchers removed the pituitary gland of mice and replaced it with a recognized to substitute of pituitary. It was found that the mouse without the pituitary gland lived longer than the mouse with the gland. It is therefore perceptible that the pituitary gland must also excrete another, unidentified, hormone that negatively affects aging. Hormonal changes are a significant part of aging. But it does not mean that hormone replacement in human beings will safely add to an individual's lifespan.

The pituitary gland produces natural HGH that is naturally stimulated by sleep and strenuous exercise. Though celluloid HGH is used in the treatment of dwarfism, not adequate research has been conducted to determine if it is risk-free to be used as an anti-aging agent.

Is the Immune System to Blame?

The rate of aging is mostly mastered by the immune system. The first body system to be compromise by normal aging is the Immune system. The master gland of the immune system, our Thymus, begins to shrink quickly with the onset of puberty. By the time we turn 40, it is only 10 to 15 per cent of the size that it was at age 11. As a result there is a decline in the production of hormones in our body.

The immune system plays a crucial role in keeping our bodies fit. Not only does it protect us against viruses and bacteria, it also helps to identify and get rid of cancer cells and toxins. Since the thymus deteriorates early, the immunity of our body is thrown out of place and the potential for elements like virus and bacteria to stimulate harm in our bodies increases.

Live Fast Die Young

The rate-of-living theory is presently the most broadly accepted explanation of aging. In ancient times, people believed that the human body degenerates in direct proportion to its use. Scientists conceive that the swiftness at which an organism breaks down oxygen is a better and precise measurement. Creatures with faster oxygen metabolic process die younger. Little mammals with rapid heartbeats metabolize oxygen quickly and have shorter lives. Tortoises, on the other hand, metabolize oxygen very slowly and have longer lives.

The rate-of-living theory of aging though helpful is not totally adequate in explaining the maximum lifetime of an organism. It has recently been discovered that the fatty acid composition of cell membranes alter consistently between species, and thereby creates variation in their metabolic rate. When the association between metabolic rate and life span was first proposed a century ago, it was not acknowledged that membrane composition varies between species.

Scientists genetically engineered mice with a defect in the hypothalamus part of the brain in order to overexert it. Since the hypothalamus of the mice was close to the temperature control centre, its brain thought the body was overheating and brought down the core temperature thereby slowing down its metabolic rate. However we do not yet know why the mice lived longer.

What we would like to know, from longevity point of view is, what decides which individuals within a species live the longest. There actually is no information that slowing down the metabolism extends human life. As a matter of fact, a slower metabolic process would put individual at risk for obesity and additional nutritional-related illnesses

Sugar and Aging Process

As we heat onions or toast bread, the sugar molecules bond to protein molecules. When this happens, a series of chemical reaction called glycation occur which results in protein molecules bonding to one another.

The same Happens in our Body but The process here is practically slower and complicated. Over time more and more protein molecules are cross-linked. These molecules do not function properly. When enough cross-linked molecules gather in a particular tissue such as cartilage, lungs, arteries and tendons, the tissues stiffen and do not function with enough efficiency this stiffening or rigidification is a symptom of growing old.

Cataracts, for example, are the rigidification of our eyes' lenses.

Although we cannot stop cross-linking, we can unquestionably slow it down. Researchers conceive that if the density of sugar in the blood is high, more cross-linking occurs. We could benefit from keeping our blood sugar from rising by avoiding foods with high glucose levels. Foods such as sweetened sodas and juices release sugar into the body quickly.

Free Radicals and Aging

Free radicals are a by-product of convention cell function. They are atoms or groups of atoms with free electrons that are formed when oxygen reacts with certain molecules. These highly reactive free electrons begin a chain of chemical reactions with significant cellular components such as DNA, or the cell membrane. This deteriorates the Cells function or even leads to the death of these cells. The body has its inbuilt defense system of antioxidants to prevent or fight the damages incurred by free radicals.

Antioxidants – The Free Radical Sponge

Antioxidants are molecules which can safely interact with free radicals and terminate the chain reaction before life-sustaining molecules are damaged. Though there are various enzyme systems within the body that clean free radicals, the principle antioxidants are vitamin E, beta-carotene, and vitamin C. Additionally, selenium, a trace metal that is compulsory for appropriate function of one of the body's antioxidant enzyme systems, is also occasionally included in the category of antioxidants.

The body cannot construct these micronutrients so it is essential that they must be catered in the diet. Antioxidants are largely found in plants. We can get the best antioxidant benefits by consuming real plants and other foods.

Several damages that take place as our body are stimulated by free radicals. These damages thus induced are known to accumulate and cause aging. Increasing the quantity of antioxidants in the diet can however slow down the consequences of aging. It is presumed that free radicals play an important role in the equation of aging.

Genetic Aging Theory

According to the genetic theory of aging, the lifetime of an individual is mostly influenced by the genes we inherit. The theory is entirely concerned with the genes in sperm and egg cells. These genes are passed down from generation to generation. Our potential age is thus chiefly decided at the moment of conception. Somatic mutations take place in the genes after we inherit them, but cannot be passed down to the offspring. Although we have evidence of gene mutations inducing damage and death of cells, it cannot be counted as the most significant factor in aging.

Mutation and Aging

A crucial part of aging is decided by what happens to our genes after we inherit them. Commencing at time of conception, our body's cells multiply continually. Each time a cell splits; some of the genes are imitated incorrectly. This is called a mutation. Exposure to toxins, radiation or ultraviolet rays can also cause mutations in our genes.

Though our body can rectify or demolish most of the chromosomal mutation, it cannot do away with them altogether. Eventually the mutated cells compile and replicate themselves and lead in problems in the functioning of the body that are associated with aging.

Chapter 2 - Is Life Extension Possible?

The term life extension deals solely with a wide mixture of approaches that aim at prolonging life. Several of these approaches are merely possibilities established on our intellect of why we age. Few, are more akin to science fiction and some may even be categorized as outright entertainment. Possibilities exist that we are capable of extending the human life to as many as 5,000 years by the end of the century by the application of biogenetics which is of course illogical. As stated above, living a healthy lifestyle and debarring risks does not ensure adding years to our life. Some of the latest theories and approaches aiming at life extension are:

Calorie Restriction

A great deal of the damage incurred due to aging in a human body is induced by the metabolism of changing food into energy. If we restrain the quantity of food intake by 30 to 50%, we can limit the damage due to aging.

Calorie limitation is a strategy established to extend a fit and maximum life span in rodents and primates. Some animal analysis carried on over the past 20 years has indicated up to a 40% increase in maximum life span. Although No studies have been completed on humans, an analysis for 6-8 years over healthy adult human beings have shown that a 20% decrease in calorie consumption relaxes conventional and disease related aging in human beings as well.

Nutritional Approaches

Catering out antioxidants and additional nutritional ingredients to the body at a greater extent will slow down the process of aging. By giving the body a lot of antioxidants, damage caused by free radicals is diminished. It is not clear whether these approaches slacken the actual aging process, or simply bring down a human being's chance of falling ill. No studies have associated these nutritional approaches with a genuine increase in life span although they are associated with a lessening in illness.

Supplements are depicted to be not as competent as consuming genuine nutrient through food. The oldest advice is still the best advice- consume good deal of Fruits and Vegetables to stay young for a longer time.

Read this brilliant book 'The Top 101 Foods that FIGHT Aging'. It gives comprehensive advice on what foods to eat to live long and healthy.

Hormone Replacement Therapy

When people age, their hormone levels, particularly human growth hormone, testosterone and DHEA worsen. Hormone-replacement therapy gives people doses of these hormones to balance the consequences and impact of aging. An individual going through hormone-replacement therapy will feel healthier for some time. But the supplements prescribed for the therapy are expected to slow down body's ability to produce these crucial hormones. Though evidence exists to associate hormone-replacement therapy with increased life span in human beings, it is definitely known to slow down the aging process.

Body Part Replacement

Some life extensionists propose that therapeutic cloning and stem cell research could one day put up a way to generate cells, body parts, or even entire bodies that would be genetically indistinguishable to a potential patient. Some even forecast the production of entire bodies, missing consciousness, for the ultimate brain transplantation.

The human body is therefore like a house, where we can replace several components but the house still remains unchanged. Disciples to this theory believe that we will be capable to develop and replace body parts as they wear out.

Cryonics

It is the low-temperature preservation of humans and animals who can no longer be kept alive by modern-day medication, with the hope that healing and resuscitation may be possible in the future. Cryonics does not believe that legal death is "real death" as though neurological damage occurs within 4–6 minutes of cardiac arrest, the permanent neurodegenerative processes do not manifest for hours.

Adherents conceive that by bringing down body temperature in a complex process that prevents freezing but chills the body to exceedingly low temperatures, one can preserve cells and tissues indefinitely. No mammal has however been successful cryo-preserved and returned to life. The common practice with us is to place a human in a cryogenic state directly upon death, but prior to the degeneration of tissues and cells. This is done in the hope that someday in the future, medication will not alone be able to resurrect an individual from this state, but also be able to treat whatsoever caused death earlier.

Chapter 3 - Hydrogen Sulfide and Longevity
- Life Extension and Hibernation

*R*esearchers at the Fred Hutchinson Cancer Research Center are trying to find out if cellular hibernation be caused by placing a chemical in our body. In order to experiment they have used Hydrogen Sulfide (H2S) to put mice into a "reverse metabolic hibernation."

Life Extension, Longevity and Hydrogen Sulfide

Research workers have detected that nematodes (tiny worms) that were raised in a controlled atmosphere with low concentrations of H2S did not hibernate. Rather, their metabolic process and reproductive activity remained normal, life span expanded and they became more tolerant to heat than untreated worms. It was found that 77% of the exposed worms lived an average of 9.6 days longer than the non-exposed ones.

Researchers believe that the hydrogen sulfide helps to regulate the SIR-2.1 gene, which is significant in longevity. When this gene is "hyperactive," it can increase the lifespan of other organisms as well by 20%. While the nematode has enough similarities with humans to be a great research example, there really isn't any evidence that living in an environment with higher hydrogen sulfide levels will extend life in humans.

H2S is normally produced in humans and animals and help regulate body temperature and metabolic activity. The chemical is similar to oxygen at the molecular level and binds many protein molecules. As a result, H2S contends for and intervenes with the body's ability to use oxygen for energy production. Researchers are excited about this course of research as a way of potentially "buying time" for critically ill patients by slowing down their metabolic process while waiting for treatment to start its effect.

Chapter 4 - Calorie Restriction and Life Extension- Cut Calories, Live Longer?

Calorie restriction is a scheme for expanding life expectancy by bringing down the total amount of calories consumed daily. Over the last 20 years there has been a rise in food consumption accompanied by an ascending incidence of obesity, cardiovascular disease and diabetes in many countries of the world. Calorie restriction research has been around since the 1930s and recent studies have demonstrated longevity benefits to rats and other animals on a low calorie diet.

In this process Calorie-poor, nutrient-dense foods such as vegetables are opted over sugars, high carbohydrate items and other foods. It is exceedingly difficult to maintain calorie restriction for long period. Consequently anyone on this diet should have knowledge on nutrition and must see their doctor for regular check-ups. On an average, while a normal American consumes between 2000 and 3000 calories per day the ones practicing calorie restriction may consume between 1500 and 2000 calories daily.

The maximum lifespan of rats has been nearly doubled in some experiments on a wholesome, low calorie diet. The advantageous effects of calorie restriction on health and life-span have also been found on other animals like monkeys, mice, and spiders. Not only do the animals on calorie restriction live longer but they also remain more youthful, energetic and healthy.

In humans, calorie restriction has been proven to lower blood pressure, improve the function of heart, veins, and arteries, and lower blood insulin levels. However it is not known if calorie restriction can increase the life expectancy in humans. However Studies over 2 – 6 years on healthy adult humans have shown that a 20% reduction in food or calorie intake slows many chances of normal and disease-related aging. Thus, it is widely believed that long-term reduction in calorie or food intake will delay the onset of age-related diseases such as heart disease, diabetes and cancer, and so prolong life.

Chapter 5 - Can Suspended Animation Extend Life?

Suspended animation is the process of slowing the life processes by foreign means without causing death. This is done through extrinsic means such as cooling the body by the use of hydrogen sulfide in accurate quantity to debar the requirement for oxygen in the body. Although breathing, heartbeat, and other involuntary functions may still take place, but they can only be perceived by artificial means.

This idea has led to all sorts of science fiction applications of suspended animation; the most common instance is the idea of stationing astronauts in suspended animation during space flights of incredibly long duration. People often get confused between suspended animation and cryonics.

In cryonics, a person is literally frozen by the use of liquid nitrogen after he has, technically, died. The proponents of cryonics believe that, as technology develops, a frozen person could be brought back to life. Some people have even opted to have their bodies frozen at the moment of death using cryonics with the hope of being brought back to life decades or centuries from now so that the cause of their death could be treated. I find the idea of Cryonics to be no other than science fiction.

Suspended animation, however, is a completely different affair. Doctors are checking up on the possibilities of placing a person in a state of suspended animation during certain surgical procedures to, in essence, buy time to mend things. Not only that, but there are other ways to accomplish suspended animation than simply cooling it. There has been research in which animals were revived after being in a "technically dead" state for three hours. If suspended animation can be developed for use in trauma and other situations, it would have the potential to increase the survival rate from these procedures.

The process of Suspended Animation bears the possibility to extend life by granting surgeons additional tools to "buy time" in order to transport patients to the place of greater care in order to grant a longer life through the success of more complex, surgical procedures.

Chapter 6 - Is Aging in Our Genes?

*W*hile some family lines have a history of smooth aging others seem to have a history of age-related ill health. But is it because the families have "good" or "bad" aging genes? Or is it because families tend to have the same behaviors and habits in each generation? There are too many possibilities and it takes too long to get information about life expectancy of human beings.

Nematodes on the other hand are an awesome research subject for aging and genetic science studies because they don't live very long and we don't have to wait a long time for results. Moreover, their genetic code is mapped and not irresistibly big.

Two types of aging are studied in aging research: chronological age and physiological age. For example, a human being can age 70, but his body may be more alike that of a 50-year-old - which is known as successful aging. Or, he may be 70 and his body functions more alike a 90-year-old -poor aging. While trying to figure out the physiological age of people is an expensive business, figuring out the physiological age of nematodes is merely research.

To test aging in worms, the research workers put the nematodes in life-threatening situations that cause the worms to react. The scientists then measured their speed, dexterity, etc. Over time, a database was assembled that depicted the average and extreme reactions of elderly nematodes. Next, researchers took all the data and looked into the DNA and genetics of the nematodes. Having a Look at genetic information alone, they could predict, the difference between the nematode's chronological age and physiological with 70% accuracy,

Am I Doomed By My Genes?

Nematodes are pretty simple beings that were matured in absolute controlled surrounds in the research laboratory. The doctrine of analogy for people would be to take people and keep them all in the one house, feed them the same nutrient and give them the equal amount of bodily function over their entire lives. A few of them will mature comfortably and others won't and we could find out who had the best genes for that environment. But we live in a world with lots of diversity. Some people might have a gene for high cholesterol that heads to heart troubles only when exposed to a poor diet but if they were on a strict vegetarian diet, this gene wouldn't embody any trouble.

The significant key is to understand the genetic factors and adapt and optimize our lifestyle to minimize risk. We aren't there yet, but await more genetic health information to appear that impacts aging. We must be prepared to make modifications to our life to accommodate a bad gene here and there. And not get too involved in all this genetics and aging talk. We know what is needed to be done to remain healthy - consume right food, exercise, de-stress, have more fun and take better rest. These are the things we can alter, our genes we can't.

Chapter 7 - New Scientific Breakthroughs – Mitochondrial and Aging

*I*s there an age limit? The longest we know that anyone has ever lived is One hundred and twenty years, Shirechiyo Izumi, a man in Japan reached the age of 120 years, 237 days in 1986. He died of pneumonia. Long lives make us wonder. It makes us question: What is the secret behind this? Does this lie in the genes? Does it depend on where people live or the way they live? Is it something they do or something they do not? Do they eat more or do they eat less? Most of the gerontologists who study aging, say that the secret probably lies in all of the above heredity, environment, and lifestyle.

But gerontologists also have other difficult questions to ask. For example, could the 120 year old have lived on and on if he had not finally succumbed to illness? Or did he approach some built-in biological limit? Is there a maximum life span beyond which we humans cannot live no matter how optimal our environment or favorable our genes are? Whether or there is such a limit not? What happens as we grow old?

What are the dynamics of the process of aging and how do they make life spans short, average or long? Once we understand these dynamics could we use them to extend everyone's life span to 120 years or more?

The most important question for us is how can we use the insights into longevity to fight the diseases and disabilities associated with old age and make sure that this period of life is healthy, active, and independent? It gives us an overview of the researches on aging and longevity, showing the major puzzle pieces already in place and to some extent provides the shapes of those that are missing.

The Genetic Connection

Scientists isolate specific genes in laboratories clone them, map them against chromosomes, and study their products to learn what they do and how they influence aging and longevity. Though Human beings seem to have a maximum life span of about 120 years, tortoises are found to live for 150 years and dogs for about 20 years. The reason for this difference is lies in specific genes- the coded segments of DNA that are strung like beads along the chromosomes of nearly every living cell.

In human beings, the nuclei of each cell holds 23 pairs of chromosomes together these 23 pairs of chromosomes contain about 100,000 genes. Therefore there is unquestioned link between genes and life span. The fact that some species have longer life spans than other species is itself a convincing piece of evidence. For example, humans live longer than dogs and tortoises longer than mice. Another piece of evidence comes from recent dramatic laboratory studies. Researchers have been able to raise animals with extended life spans through selective breeding and genetic engineering. For example, fruit flies bred through selective breeding have lived nearly twice as long as average flies.

Longevity Genes

The longer-lived fruit flies have set the stage for more questions by certifying that genes are associated to life span. What are specific genes involved in this process? What is it that sparks off them? How do these genes regulate aging and longevity? The search for answers is on in a number of research laboratories around the world.

We have found some leads from yeast cells where research workers have detected the evidence of 14 genes that appear to be associated to aging. Longevity-related genes have also been found in tiny worms called nematodes and fruit flies. Nematodes and fruit flies Like yeast, have short life spans and their genes, which are recognized and do not vary greatly are easier to examine.

In the Lab of the Long-Lived Fruit Flies

A Research laboratory in the University of California, Irvine, constitutes the abode of thousands of Drosophila melanogaster or fruit flies that live for 70 or 80 days. This is nearly double the lifespan of an average Drosophila melanogaster. The evolutionary biologist, Michael Rose has bred these flies by choosing and mating the flies late in life.

To begin with the process of genetic selection, Rose first collected the eggs lay by middle-aged female fruit flies and then let them hatch in isolation. The offspring were later shifted to a communal Plexiglas cage to consume, develop, and multiply under conditions ideal for mating. Once they had reached an advanced age, the eggs laid by aged females that were fertilized by aged males were once again collected and removed to separate hatching vials. Though the cycle was repeated, yet, the day on which the eggs were collected was increasingly delayed with succeeding generations. After 15 such generations (two years approx) the research laboratory had a breed of Drosophila melanogaster with longer life spans.

The question that follows up is what are the genes and gene products that are involved? Since the first experiment, Rose has bred longer life spans into fruit flies by choosing for additional features, such as power to resist starving, so the flies' long life spans are not need fully attached to their fertility late in life.

One possible action is that the anti-oxidant enzyme, SOD is involved. In another research laboratory at Irvine, the late Robert Tyler had discovered that the longer-lived flies had a fairly different form of the SOD gene, which was more active than its counterpart in the flies with average life spans. This discovery has yielded an encouragement to the hypothesis that anti-oxidant enzymes like SOD are associated to aging or longevity.

Some of the genes found in yeast and fruit flies appear to encourage long life spans while others may even reduce it. One such "death gene" has been detached from nematodes' genes by research workers at the University of Colorado. Here it was establish that chromosomal mutation of a certain chromosome can increase the life span by more than double of the nematode's normal 3-week life span.

Thomas Johnson's laboratory in Boulder has also exposed evidence that the mutant might extend life span by overproducing super oxide dismutase (SOD) and catalase, the two anti-oxidant enzymes that have been associated to longevity in various additional studies as well.

These genes detached as yet are only some of what scientists believe might constitute dozens, perhaps hundreds, of longevity and aging-related genes. Tracking these genes down in organisms like nematodes and yeast is merely the beginning. The next big question for many gerontologists is whether there are similitudes of these aging genes in people, as human homologous similitudes of the genes found in research laboratory animals.

Additional unanswered doubts are associated to the roles played by these genes. What precisely do the genes do? On one degree, all genes function by transcribing their "codes". These codes are deoxyribonucleic acid base sequences that are recorded into a different nucleic acid called messenger ribonucleic acid or messenger RNA. The Messenger RNA is then transformed into proteins. Thus Transcription and translation together comprise the process known as gene expression. The proteins so conveyed by genes execute a large number of roles in each cell and tissue of the body, where a few of the roles are related to aging. So when we inquire what longevity or aging-related genes do, we are in reality asking what their protein products do at the cellular and tissue layers.

Increasingly, gerontologists also ask how adjustments in the process of gene expression itself may affect aging. Some proteins, such as anti-oxidants, prevent damage to cells, and others might amend damaged deoxyribonucleic acid or aid cells react to stress. Other gene products are believed to master cell senescence, which is a process that could prove to be a key piece in the puzzle of aging and longevity.

Cell Senescence

A cell has threadlike pairs of chromosomes that inhabit a nucleus which floats in a sea of cytoplasm along with other tiny organelles that do the cell's work. This whole thing is surrounded by a membrane at the surface of which the cell sends and receives messages from other cells. Now, let us see what chromosomes are. Chromosomes are condensed rod-like structures that divide in two during cell division. Then the nucleus disappears and the chromosomes migrate to opposite sides of the cell where nuclei are formed. After this, the entire cell follows the chromosomes and pull apart to form two identical daughter cells. This process of mitosis or asexual cell division takes place in about all of the 100 trillion approximately cells that comprise the human body. But the process doesn't go on indefinitely. The research workers have discovered that cells have limited life spans at least when analyzed in test tubes - in vitro.

An inbuilt limit in cellular division may help oneself explain the aging process. After a certain number of divisions, the cells enter a state of cell senescence, in which they don't split or proliferate and deoxyribonucleic acid synthesis is barred.

For instance, young human fibroblasts collagen-producing cells that are frequently used in this branch of aging research are found to divide about 50 times and then stop. This phenomenon has come to be known as the Hayflick limit, after Leonard Hayflick, who first described it with Paul Moorhead at the Wistar Institute in Philadelphia. Fascinated by the possibility that the Hayflick limit might be competent to aid in explaining some aspects of corporeal aging, gerontologists have sought and found links between senescence and human life spans. Fibroblasts taken from 75-year-old human beings, for instance, have fewer divisions left than cells taken from a child. Moreover, the longer a species' life span is, the higher is its Hayflick limit. Therefore human fibroblasts have higher Hayflick limits than mice fibroblasts.

Proliferative Genes

While looking for explanations of proliferation and senescence, scientists have detected certain genes that seem to trigger cell proliferation. One good example of such a Proliferative gene is c-fos, which ciphers a short-lived protein that governs the manifestation of other genes crucial in cellular division. But c-fos and others of its variety are forced to clash certain anti-Proliferative genes, which appear to intervene with cellular division. The first evidence of an anti-Proliferative gene came from an eye tumor called retinoblastoma.

When one of the genes from retinoblastoma cells (which were later called the RB gene) became suspended, the cells went on dividing indefinitely and developed tumor. But when the RB gene product was activated, the cells arrested dividing. This gene's product, in other words, appeared to suppress proliferation.

Senescence is the norm in the world of cells. In some cases, however, a cell somehow breaks loose this control mechanism and goes on dividing thereby becoming immortal in terms of cell biology. And since immortal cells eventually form tumors, this is where aging research and cancer research intersect. Researchers speculate that a failure of anti-Proliferative genes which is also known as tumor suppressor gene is the first step in a complex process that leads to growth of a tumor. Senescence, according to this view, may have developed because it fortified us from cancer.

Mystery lies in how these genes operate to boost and curb cell proliferation. There are indications that a multi layer control system is already active. This in all probability involves a host of intricate mechanisms that interact to sustain a balance between the two varieties of genes. Many gerontologists are now involved in untangling these intricacies, analyzing both the genes and their products to find out which ones regulate senescence and how.

Tracking Down a Longevity Gene

Investigators are trying to finding out clues to aging and longevity in yeast, one-celled organisms that have some challenging genetic similarities to human cells. In a laboratory at Louisiana State University Medical Center in New Orleans, Michal Jazwinski has detected genes that seem to boost longevity in these rapidly splitting, easy-to-study beings. Yeast generally has approximately 21 cell divisions or generations. Jazwinski discovered that over the flow of that "life span," certain genes in the yeast are more dynamic or less dynamic as the cells age; in the language of molecular biology, they're differentially conveyed.

Hitherto, Jazwinski has witnessed 14 such genes in yeast. Choosing one of these genes, Jazwinski attempted two different experiments. First, he inserted the gene into yeast cells in a form that permitted him to check its activity. When the gene was activated to a greater level than average, or over expressed, a few of the yeast cells went on dividing for 27 or 28 generations; their period of activity was broadened by 30 percent.

In his second experiment, Jazwinski mutated the gene. While he introduced this non-working edition into a group of yeast cells, they had only approximately 12 divisions. The two experiments made it clear that the gene, now called LAG-1, regulates the number of divisions in yeast or, according to some research worker*' ways of thinking, its longevity. (LAG-1 is short for longevity assurance gene.) But how it acts is still a mystery. One little clue dwells in its sequence of deoxyribonucleic acid bases -- its genetic code -- which proposes that it produces a protein found in cell membranes. One next step comprises the survey of the function of that protein. Similar sequences have been detected in human being deoxyribonucleic acid, so a second investigatory path is to clone the human gene and analyze its function. If there turns out to be a human LAG-1 counterpart, fresh insights into aging may be revealed.

Telomeres

Meanwhile, scientists have discovered additional clues to senescence in the architecture of deoxyribonucleic acid. Every chromosome, they've detected, has tails at the ends that become shorter when a cell splits. Named telomeres, the tails all have the identical, brief sequence of DNA bases duplicated thousands of times. The repetitive structure steadies the chromosomes, constituting a compressed bonding between the two strands of the deoxyribonucleic acid. Each time a cell splits, the telomeres shed a number of bases, so telomere length gives roughly indication of how many divisions the cell has already undergone and how many remain before it turns senescent.

This visible calculating mechanism, almost like an abacus holding course of the cell's age, has led to supposition that telomeres do serve as molecular meters of cellular division. But they might play a more participating function, and telomere investigators are researching the possibility that these chromosome ends govern cellular life span somehow. The duplicated deoxyribonucleic acid bases in telomeres form close bonds that assist stabilize chromosomes. About 50 bases are misplaced from each telomere every time a convention cell divides.

Telomere research is a different territory where cancer and aging research blend. In immortal cancer cells, telomeres behave abnormally -- they stop contracting with each cell division. In the hunt for hints to this phenomenon, investigators have zeroed in on an enzyme called telomerase. Commonly absent in mature cells, telomerase seems to swing into action in advanced cancers, enabling the telomeres to substitute lost sequences and split indefinitely. This discovery has headed to speculation that if a drug could be formulated to bar telomerase activity, it might help in cancer treatment.

Whether cell senescence is explained by abnormal gene products, telomere reducing, or additional factors, the question of what senescence has to do with the aging of organisms continues and remains to be the focus of acute analyze. In the meantime, gerontologists are also analyzing proteins in the body that might play a purpose in aging and longevity.

Genes bind the codes to these proteins, but what substances turn the genes off and on? And once triggered, how do their products interact with the products of a different genes? What is their impression on cells and tissues? The biochemistry of aging gives some of the solutions.

Biochemistry and Aging

Proteins, in their countless forms and functions, are the substances most responsible the daily functioning of living beings. A few of these proteins appear to impact the way we mature and how long we live. Unreliable oxygen molecules, protective enzymes, hormones that appear to turn back the clock, and proteins that might accelerate it up: The biochemistry of aging is a fertile dominion with an expanding frontier. Major areas of exploration include oxygen radicals and glucose cross linking of proteins, both of which harm cells; the essences that help prevent and amend damage; and the role of particular proteins, especially heat shock proteins, hormones, and development agents.

Oxygen Radicals

Tearing down proteins and damaging nucleic acids, oxygen radicals are believed to be the villains in the every day life of cells. The free radical theory of aging, first proposed by Denham Harman at the University of Nebraska, holds that damage induced by oxygen radicals is responsible for a lot of the physical changes that accompany aging.

Free radicals have been involved not only in aging but also in chronic disorders, including cancer, atherosclerosis, cataracts, and neuro degeneration. They damage cells and might cause tissues and organs to age. A free radical is a molecule with an unpaired, extremely unstable electron. An oxygen-free radical is a by-product of convention metabolic process, produced as cells turn food and oxygen into energy.

In need of a pair for its solitary electron, the free radical accepts an electron from a different molecule, which in turn becomes unstable and combines promptly with other molecules. A chain reaction can ensue, resulting in a series of chemical compound*, some of which are harmful. They damage proteins, tissue layer*, and nucleic acids, especially deoxyribonucleic acid, including the DNA in mitochondria, the organelles inside the cell that create energy.

But free radicals do not go unrestrained. Mounted against them is a multi layer defense system manned by anti-oxidants that react with and disarm these destructive molecules. Anti-oxidants include nutrients -- the familiar vitamins C and E and beta carotene -- as well as enzymes, such as super oxide dismutase (SOD), catalase, and glutathione peroxides. They prevent almost, but not completely, oxidative damage. By small degrees the damage mounts and contributes, so the possibility goes, to deteriorating tissues and organs.

Support for the free radical theory comes from studies of anti-oxidants, especially SOD. SOD converts oxygen radicals into the also adverse hydrogen peroxide, which is then degraded by a different enzyme, catalase, to oxygen and water.

Anti-Oxidants and Aging Gerbils

An encouragement for the theory that high degrees of anti-oxidants can slacken the aging process descends from an analysis of N-tert-butyl-alpha-phenylnitrone or PBN in gerbils. Though it does not occur naturally in the body, PBN works in a good deal the same method as beta-carotene and other anti-oxidants by adhering and neutralizing free radicals.

Older gerbils had been shown to have enhanced levels of oxidized protein in their brains by two researchers, Robert A. Floyd at the Oklahoma Medical Research Foundation and John M. Carney at the University of Kentucky. Curious about the consequences of anti-oxidants in elderly animals,

Floyd and Carney organized an experiment to learn whether PBN could bring down oxidized protein levels in gerbils' brains. Over a time period of 14 days they applied PBN to two groups of gerbils, one comprised of young grownups, the other of older grownups.

As the older gerbils were treated with PBN, their degrees of oxidized protein diminished until they were nearly comparable to degrees detected in the younger animals. After treatment ended, oxidized protein gradually returned to pretreatment levels. PBN made no effect on the young gerbils.

Although it is only one analyze and more are needed, this investigation affirms the idea that maintaining anti-oxidant defense levels may be vital during aging. It also suggests that interference such as PBN might someday provide the means.

At the National Institute on Aging (NIA), Richard Cutler has detected that SOD levels are straightaway related to life span in 20 different species; longer-lived animals have higher levels of SOD, suggesting that the ability to fight free radicals has something to do with longer life spans. Levels of other anti-oxidants -- vitamin E and beta-carotene, for instance -- have also been related with life span.

Other studies have shown that introducing additional copies of the SOD gene into fruit flies expands their average life span. In three different research laboratory*, researchers have described that transgenic fruit flies, bearing extra copies of the gene for SOD, live 5 to 10 percent longer than average.

Other observational evidence lends support to the free radical possibility. For example, higher levels of SOD and catalase have been detected in long-lived nematodes. And in another important analyze, giving gerbils a celluloid anti-oxidant has cut down high levels of oxidized protein, a mark of aging, in their brains.

The discovery of anti-oxidants called forth hopes that people could slow down aging merely by adding them to the diet. Unfortunately taking SOD tablets induces no impression on cellular aging; the enzyme is merely broken down in the body during digestion. And when anti-oxidant vitamins are added to cells, they make up by arresting production of their own anti-oxidants, leaving free radical levels unaltered.

Researchers have not given up all hope for dietary anti-oxidants, however. Current studies are researching the possibility that vitamin C can reduce heart disease by barring oxidation of low-density lipoproteins. Oxidation of these cholesterol-carrying proteins is believed to comprise a key element in hardening of the arteries. In addition, there is evidence that vitamin E in the diet may be linked to heart attacks, with low vitamin E intake coming along to increase the risk.

Glucose Cross linking

Another suspect in cellular impairment is blood sugar or glucose. In a process called non-enzymatic glycosylation or glycation, glucose molecules bind themselves to proteins, launching a chain of chemical reactions that ends in the proteins adhering together or cross linking, thus changing their biological and structural roles. The process is slow but gains with time.

Cross links, which have been termed advanced glycosylation end products (AGEs), appear to toughen tissues and may cause some of the impairment associated with aging. AGEs have been linked to rigidifying connective tissue (collagen), hardened arteries, clouded eyes, loss of nerve function, and less efficient kidneys.

These are inadequacies that often come with aging. They also come along at younger ages in people with diabetes, who have high glucose levels. Diabetes, is sometimes regarded an accelerated model of aging. Not only do its ramifications mimic the physiologic changes that can accompany old age, but its victims have shorter life expectancies. As a result, much research on cross linking has concentrated on its relationship to diabetes as well as aging.

One happy encountering is that the body has its own defense system against cross linking. Just as it has anti-oxidants to fight free-radical impairment, it has other guardians, immune system cells called macrophages that combat glycation. Macrophages with special sensory receptors for AGEs seek them out, engulf them, break them down, and discharge them into the blood stream where they are strained out by the kidneys and got rid of in urine.

Glucose, which is the basic reservoir of energy, reacts with and cross-linking essential molecules and the only evident drawback to this defense system is that it is not complete and levels of AGEs gain steadily with age. One reason is that kidney function tends to fall with advancing age.

Another is that macrophages, like certain other elements of the immune system, become less active agent. Why is not known, but immunologists are commencing to learn more about how the immune system affects and is affected by aging. And in the meantime, diabetes investigators are investigating drugs that could add on the body's natural defenses by blocking AGE constitution.

Cross linking interests gerontologists for various reasons. It is linked with disorders that are common among aged people, such as diabetes; it advances with age; and AGEs are likely targets for anti-aging drugs. In addition, cross linking might play a purpose in damage to DNA, which has become another significant focus for research on aging.

DNA Repair

In the normal depreciation of cellular life, DNA undergoes continuous damage. Attacked by oxygen radicals, ultraviolet light, and other toxic agents, it endures damage in the form of omissions, or ruined segments, and genetic mutation*, or changes in the sequence of DNA bases that comprise the genetic code.

Biologists suppose that this DNA damage, which gradually gathers, leads to malfunctioning genes, proteins, cells, and, as the years go by, degenerating tissues and organs. Not surprisingly, numerous enzyme systems in the cell have evolved to detect and repair battered DNA.

The repair operation interests gerontologists. It is known that an animal's ability to repair certain types of DNA impairment is directly associated to the life span of its species. Human beings repair DNA, for instance, more promptly and with efficiency than mice or other animals with shorter life spans. This suggests that DNA impairment and repair are somehow part of the aging puzzle.

Additionally, researchers have found faults in DNA repair in people with a genetic or hereditary susceptibility to cancer. If DNA repair operations decline with age while damage compiles, as scientists hypothesize, it could help explain why cancer is so very much more common amongst older people.

Gerontologists who study DNA impairment and repair have begun to expose numerous complexities. Even within a single being, repair rates can alter among cells, with the most effective repair going on in terms (sperm and egg) cell. Furthermore, certain genes are amended more quickly than others, including those that govern cell proliferation.

Frontiers

Gerontology is channels toward a deeper intellect of aging in the search for ways to make it a fitter process.

New territory, undiscovered or only sketchily represented, lies ahead. As gerontologists set apart and qualify more and more longevity- and aging-related genes in research laboratory animals, insights into genes and gene products important in human aging will come forth. Parallel human genes will be discovered and mapped to chromosomes.

This data will be valuable in planning both genetic and non-genetic interferences to slow or even reverse some aging-related alterations. Already, for example, a analyze by Helen Blau of Stanford University has shown that muscle cells can be genetically altered and injected into muscle where they will develop and secrete human growth hormone.

Non-genetic strategies include the evolution of interferences to reduce damage to cellular elements, such as proteins, nucleic acids, and lipids.

Convention aging will be more intimately defined. For instance, at NIA's Gerontology Research Center, the conduct of the cells that line blood vessels during aging is now furnishing clues to the rigidification of blood vessels that comes with age as well as insights into vascular disease. As key biomarkers of aging are identified, researchers will be able to use them to test interventions to slow aging. Analyses will begin to dig more deeply into differences in aging between the genders and among cultural groups.

In short, gerontologists will be charting the paths and overlaps of genetic, biochemical, and physiological aging. What they find will reveal some of the mysteries of aging. It may lead to prolonged life spans. It will very certainly contribute to fuller health, lower impairment, and more independence in the second fifty years of life.

Chapter 8 - Aging Glossary

Anti-oxidants – These are compounds that neutralize free oxygen radicals. A few of them are enzymes like SOD while others are nutrients such as vitamin C, vitamin E, and beta-carotene. High levels of anti-oxidants have been associated with longer life spans.

Anti-proliferate genes - Genes that suppress cell division or proliferation; also known as tumor suppressor genes

Average life span - The average number of years that members of a population live.

Biomarkers- Biological alterations that characterize the aging process; because biomarkers are considered a better measure of aging than chronological time, studies are afoot to identify biomarkers in cells, tissues, and organs.

Caloric restriction – It is an experimental approach to study longevity in which the life span of research laboratory animals have been extended by bringing down their calorie intake but the level of nutrition is maintained.

Cell senescence – It is the stage at which cells stop dividing permanently.

Chromosomes – They are anatomical structures in a cell's nucleus that are made up of protein and DNA that carry the genes.

DNA (deoxyribonucleic acid) – It is a large molecule that bears all the genetic information essential for cellular functions, including the construction of proteins. The rate of damage in DNA helps us in determining the rate of aging.

Free radicals – They are molecules with odd free electrons that react promptly with other molecules. Oxygen-free radicals produced during metabolic process damage cells and may cause aging in tissues and organs.

Gene – It is a segment of DNA that contains the "code" for a particular protein.

Gene expression – It is the process by which genes are transcribed and changed into proteins. Age-related alterations in genes may account for some of the phenomena of aging.

Glycation – It is the process by which glucose links with proteins and causes them to bind together.

It leads to stiffening tissues and heading to the complications of diabetes and perhaps some of the physiological problems that are associated to aging.

Hay flick limit –It is the limited number of times that cells are capable of dividing.

Interleukins –They are the substances that are secreted by lymphocytes. The level of secretion however varies with age.

Lymphocytes – They are small white blood cells (WBC) that are important to the immune system. A decline in lymphocyte functions with increasing age insights into aging and disease.

Maximum life span - The maximum age reached by a member of any given species.

Mitochondria - Cell organelles that metabolize sugar into energy. They also contain DNA which is damaged by the high amount of free radicals produced in the mitochondria.

Proliferate genes – They are genes that promote cell division or proliferation. They are also known as transforming gene.

Photo-aging – It is the process started by sunlight by which the skin becomes drier and loses elasticity. Photo-aging has the same effect as normal aging on certain skin cells.

Proteins – They are Molecules built of amino acid arranged in a particular order that is determined by the genetic code. Proteins play an essential role in all life processes. Some of the protein molecules, such as the enzymes that protect against free radicals and the lymphocytes produced in the immune system is being studied extensively by gerontologists.

PS: I hope you enjoyed reading the book and found it beneficial. I will appreciate if you will please review the book for benefit of the other readers. .

About The Author

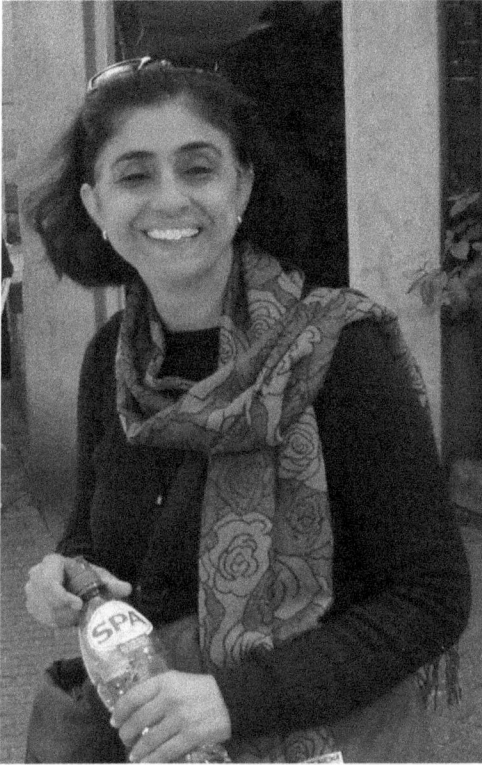

*R*achita Kumar is Bachelor of Science in Nutrition and Child Psychology. Since leaving college she has been keenly interested in science of anti-aging and how by eating correct foods you can slow the aging process in the body and skin. She writes books and articles on anti-aging, nutrition, health and women's issues.

For more information on anti-aging, nutrition and health issues visit her website http://healthywisechoice.com

Rachita's husband Praveen is an investor, business builder and a best-selling author who has helped hundreds of people to get started on their journey to create sustainable wealth with minimum risk.

You can skype Praveen Kumar on **'praveenkumar444'**